Dr. Goiz'

MEDICAL BIOMAGNETIC PAIR THERAPY

AND

BIOENERGETICS MADE EASY

Frequently Asked Questions To
Discover, Empower And Get Results

MOSES DURAZO

ISBN: 9798392712731
Independently published

Previous Title: *How You Can Prevent, Improve and Cure Disease Using Magnets - Goizean Medical Biomagnetism & Bioenergetics Frequently Asked Questions*

Meet the Author at: *www.SaveMeMagnets.com*

With a heart full of gratitude, I dedicate this book to my beloved parents, Arturo and Teresa. Their unwavering love and constant support have been the driving force behind all my achievements in life. From a young age, they instilled in me a deep curiosity and a hunger for knowledge, answering as best they could my endless questions about the world around us. They never hesitated to push me to find answers on my own and encouraged me to use my knowledge to help others. Their guidance and unwavering belief in me has been the cornerstone of my success in the field of Biomagnetism. I am forever indebted to them for all the encouragement, guidance, and support they have provided me throughout my journey. Dad, although you are no longer physically with me, your presence is very much felt in every aspect of my life, and I know that your love and blessings continue to guide me. Thank you, Mom and Dad, for everything.

DISCLAIMER

Contents

INTRODUCTION....9
SUCCESS STORIES USING MEDICAL PAIR BIOMAGNETISM....13
FOR WHOM IS MEDICAL BIOMAGNETISM INTENDED?....17
Can Biomagnetism Help me if I don't have problems?....18
Is Biomagnetism invasive?....18
Is Biomagnetism preventative?....19
What kind of equipment is used?....20
Who discovered Medical Pair Biomagnetism?....20
Is there scientific evidence?....21
Despite the evidence, why is there skepticism?....22
The difference between *Magnet Therapy, Medical Biomagnetism* and *Recalibration Biomagnetism?*....23
BIOMAGNETIC SCIENCE AND PH- IMBALANCE-CAUSING FACTORS....25
What can Biomagnetism cure?....26
What causes pH imbalances?....27
What is a: virus, bacteria, fungus or a parasite?....27
What are dysfunctions?....28
What are toxins?....29
What is a psychological disorder?....30
What are emotional challenges?....30
What are deficiencies?....31

What is spirituality and spiritual interference? 32
What is a foreign DNA? 33
What is a malignancy? 33
What are Chakra imbalances? 34
What is a reservoir? 34
How do you detect specific pH distortions? 34
What is Bioenergetics? 35
Do I need to believe for it to work? 36
SAFETY AND CONTRAINDICATIONS 37
How old must you be to try Medical Biomagnetism? 38
Is Biomagnetism safe for pregnant women? 38
Is Biomagnetism safe while on chemotherapy or other treatments? 38
Is Biomagnetism painful? 39
What happens when I mix Biomagnetism with allopathic treatment? 39
Does Biomagnetism interfere with other natural therapies? 40
Does Biomagnetism interfere with metallic surgical implants? ..40
Does Biomagnetism interfere with pacemakers? 40
WHAT TO EXPECT ON YOUR VISITS 41
What is the Private Membership Medical Association document? 41
What is the symptom questionnaire? 42
What is the initial interview like? 43
How long are the sessions? 43
What if I can't lie down for a long time? 44
Can somebody come with me to my appointment? 44
What will I feel during the biomagnetic session? 45
What did you find? What's wrong with me? 45
How did I get this condition/infection/problem? 45
What will I feel after the biomagnetic session? 46
What is a healing crisis? 46

What if I don't feel anything after my session? 47
What should I do after a session? 48
SPECIAL SERVICES:
MAGNO-GUIDE AND DISTANCE HEALING 49
What is Distance Healing? 51
Can I treat my pet with Biomagnetism? 51
THE BIG ISSUES 53
Can you guarantee a cure? 53
How many sessions do I need? 53
How much does it cost, and does insurance pay for it? 54
Should I go to the hospital or do Biomagnetism first? 54
Do you prescribe medication or supplements? 54
Should I stop taking medication or supplements? 55
Are there people who cannot be helped? 55
Can I put magnets on myself? 56
BONUS SELF-CARE STRATEGY:
THREE MAGNETS FOR PAIN RELIEF 57
Suggested for: 57
CONCLUSION 61
ABOUT THE AUTHOR MOSES DURAZO 63
WORKS CITED 65

INTRODUCTION

THIS BOOK IS NOT just another book, but a question-and-answer guide designed to help you take back control of your health and achieve optimal energy. My goal with this and all other books I have published are to inspire you to think differently about your health, treatments, self-care, and to introduce you to alternative ways to achieve optimal well-being.

The statistics are alarming. Conventional allopathic medicine, with its heavy reliance on drugs, surgery, and technology, is now the third leading cause of death in the United States according to conservative figures. The non-conservative statistics show that allopathic medicine is perhaps the number one leading cause of death in the US because deaths may go unreported for fear of lawsuits and in other cases because codes for medication drug side-effects and other medical errors may not exist. The treatments prescribed by the allopathic medical system are often inefficient and sometimes as harmful as the disease itself. This has resulted in millions of people living with a diminished quality of life, and in some cases premature death.

Because the governments of the world have given the allopathic medical system, the pharmaceutical industry, public health agencies, big tech, the media and their cohorts the authorization to dictate what constitutes valid or effective treatments, as a whole we are very much misled through fear-mongering propaganda to believe that no other solutions exists except those of the classical doctor.

Their message is one of arrogance and danger, asserting that pharmacology reigns supreme over our body's natural intelligence and its capacity for self-healing. They dismiss other God-given natural remedies and resources as ineffective or feeble and brand them as quackery and misinformation. Those in power relentlessly censor and spread false information about anything that does not align with their beliefs.

If the authorities in medicine have, and continue to fail us when it comes to prevention, improving and curing our illness, then who, what, when, where, and how do we find the solution(s)?

The good news is that there are natural mind-body lifestyle solutions available to help you achieve balance and optimal health. More and more people are seeking wellness care as opposed to emergency, pain, and suffering care. In fact, 62% of the adult US population uses alternative medicines each year, and that number is growing.

One of the most successful natural medicine modalities gaining recognition for its efficacy in helping people prevent, improve, and cure disease is *Goizean Medical Pair Biomagnetism* (as a tribute to Dr. Isaac Goiz Duran, M.D. who discovered this science), and is also known as the *Biomagnetic Pair* or *Medical Biomagnetism.* This natural treatment uses magnetic energy and has helped men, women, and children of all ages overcome a wide variety of ailments without medication, and thus improving their quality of life. People have even been cured of cancers, asthma, lupus, arthritis, and much more.

This book will give you answers to many questions about how this therapy can help you and your family obtain an increased quality of life. My hope is that rather than waiting on approval by the conventional medical system and the pharmaceutical complex that controls the deficient medical narrative, that you have the courage to integrate the safe, natural, powerful and practical Goizean Medical Pair Biomagnetism into your own treatment plans as a primary option, whether for current health challenges or used for prevention and maintenance care.

If you want to start using a simplified self-care biomagnetic therapy approach, we suggest making the ultimate *Biomagnetic Recalibration System* or any of the quick start biomagnetic kits. Undoubtedly, these self-care tools and strategies belong in your home wellness cabinet as they provide immediate strategies for you to optimize the quality of your life. You may find more information about these self-care biomagnetic kits, courses and wellness challenges by visiting *www.SaveMeMagnets.com*.

I urge you to take control of your health, and to explore the many natural medicine options available to you. I hope this book helps you make an informed decision about this powerful transformational science called Medical Biomagnetism and helps you make it a part of your life together with the self-care Recalibration Biomagnetism strategies.

SUCCESS STORIES USING MEDICAL PAIR BIOMAGNETISM

THE POWER OF MEDICAL Biomagnetism to improve health and quality of life is demonstrated in the following success stories. These cases show the effectiveness of this therapy in treating a wide range of conditions, from diabetes and inflammation to eye sight and aggression.

In one case, a man in his 50's with diabetes reported feeling bloated and constantly annoyed with everyone. After just four medical biomagnetic pair treatments, he felt much better, and his ophthalmologist noticed a 5% improvement in his eyesight, which is *"unusual under the circumstances,"* said that doctor.

In another case, a 13-year-old girl had warts on all 10 fingers and her upper lip, which had previously been treated by freezing them off with liquid nitrogen, but they grew back even bigger. After just one week of only one biomagnetic pair treatment, the warts started to shrink, and within 30 days, they had all disappeared.

Biomagnetism has also been effective in treating infertility and pregnancy-related issues. In one case, a woman who had not had a menstrual period in seven years had a period after just one treatment and became pregnant a few months later. In another case, a woman with an ovarian cyst that put her at high risk of miscarriage stopped bleeding within hours of her initial biomagnetic pair treatment, and the cyst eventually disappeared.

Chronic pain is another area where Biomagnetism has shown remarkable results. One man suffering from back pain for over 22 years found relief after just four biomagnetic sessions, and he also lost a lot of weight. Another man with arthritis pain had an 80% reduction in pain after just one treatment, leading him to stop taking medication and improving his sleep and digestion.

Despite my many years in the medical biomagnetic healing field, I still find myself amazed by the results I witness, including cases where surgeries are avoided altogether. One example involves a woman who was scheduled for pancreatic surgery in just two weeks' time. After receiving a second biomagnetic session a week later, her chronic vomiting ceased. Further medical testing revealed that she was actually in good health and the surgery was no longer necessary. Another woman diagnosed with breast cancer underwent Medical Biomagnetism for three months before her scheduled mastectomy. When the surgeon evaluated her, there was no sign of a tumor, and the surgery was canceled. She did not require chemotherapy afterward.

In some cases, Biomagnetism has even been effective in treating terminal illnesses. In one case, a man diagnosed with terminal bone cancer had an increase in the quality of his life, experiencing less pain, more optimism, and making a strong effort to care for himself during his final days.

Finally, even minor improvements can have a significant impact on quality of life. In one case, a woman noticed only minor changes in her body after two to three biomagnetic pair treatments, but her blood pressure became normal for the first time in over a decade, leading to a reduction in medication dosage and eventually discontinuation.

These success stories demonstrate the power of Medical Biomagnetism to improve health and quality of life, even in cases where conventional medicine has failed. While 100% cures may not always happen, improvement is always possible. Even in terminal cases, increased quality of life is seen as healing, and we hope that these success stories inspire others to take action towards better health.

FOR WHOM IS MEDICAL BIOMAGNETISM INTENDED?

TO TRULY UNDERSTAND THE power of Medical Biomagnetism, we must first understand the common problems it can solve. If you and your family are feeling constantly tired, in pain, or frustrated with the limitations of conventional medicine, then Medical Biomagnetism may be the solution you have been searching for.

This natural medical science utilizes magnets to bring biochemical balance to our bodies, promoting optimal health and preventing disease. It is a natural solution that can help the body obtain homeostasis which may lead to curing conditions, but it is also effective for healthy people who want to maintain balance and prevent disease.

It is important to note that while exercise and a balanced diet are crucial for maintaining good health, they are not always enough to prevent illness. Even those that believe they are healthy individuals can be diagnosed with serious illnesses like cancer, arthritis, or diabetes. This is where Medical Biomagnetism can provide hope, healing, prevention and optimization.

If you have been diagnosed with a debilitating condition, or if you are concerned about your health in the future, medical biomagnetic therapy may be the answer. With just a few sessions, you can experience the transformative power of Biomagnetism for yourself.

If you are skeptical, you are not alone. But the truth is you will never know what is possible until you try it. This book is designed to help you understand the science behind Medical Biomagnetism and take action to improve your health and quality of life. You can even learn how to perform self-care Biomagnetism on yourself through the biomagnetic formulas in our self-care Biomagnetic Recalibration System.

Don't let pain, illness, or frustration control your life any longer. With Biomagnetism, you can take control of your health and live your life to the fullest.

Can Biomagnetism help me if I don't have problems?

Biomagnetism is not only for those who have symptoms or diagnoses, but it is also for healthy individuals who want to maintain optimal health and prevent future diseases. Even if you feel fine, there may be silent diseases that you are not aware of that can progress and harm your health.

While conventional medical testing and check-ups are important, they do not always catch everything. Many people still experience heart attacks, strokes, and other health crises despite having regular medical attention. This is where Biomagnetism comes in as both a primary and even complementary approach to health care. It helps identify and correct pH imbalances before they turn into symptoms or diagnoses.

Is Biomagnetism invasive?

Unlike invasive allopathic medical procedures, Biomagnetism is a non-invasive practice that does not require you to undress or consume medication or supplements. You remain fully clothed, and the magnets are placed over your clothes. The practitioner only needs to hold your shoes briefly to measure your leg length. Moreover, you do not have to reveal any personal information or emotional challenges that you are not ready to share. The focus is solely on the body's DNA decoding the practitioner's questions and identifying (diagnosing) where the magnets need to be placed to facilitate healing.

If you are interested in exploring Biomagnetism, you can start with a self-care kit from www.SaveMeMagnets.com. Biomagnetism is a partnership that supports your health goals and helps restore your inner balance, allowing you to achieve whatever you are ready for in life.

Is Biomagnetism preventative?

Biomagnetism offers a unique approach to healthcare that prioritizes balance and prevention. Health challenges can be difficult to detect and often go unnoticed until they become more severe. Germs, stress, and aging are inevitable factors that can lead to disease, but we can take proactive steps to prevent these issues from getting worse. By incorporating Biomagnetism, it may help erase biochemical distortions and achieve a state of balance, so that your body can function optimally and better fight off illness.

In addition to physical health benefits, Biomagnetism can also have a positive impact on emotional well-being. When we are emotionally balanced, we are better equipped to handle life's challenges with confidence and resilience. By taking control of our health and well-being, we can enjoy a richer, more fulfilling life free of pain and suffering.

It is important to remember that prevention is key when it comes to healthcare. By prioritizing our physical and emotional health, we can ensure that we are better equipped to handle whatever life throws our way. So why not give Biomagnetism a try? Incorporating this natural solution into your daily routine may just be the key to achieving optimal health and wellness.

What kind of equipment is used?

Biomagnetism is a natural therapy that uses static magnets to help restore the balance of the body's biochemistry. The magnets used in Biomagnetism are permanent magnets, similar to refrigerator magnets but much stronger.

It is important to note that Biomagnetism does not use electrical currents or potentially harmful electromagnetism. When it comes to the strength and materials of the magnets used, Biomagnetism practitioners use magnets that are a minimum of 1,000 Gauss in strength for therapeutic purposes. Magnets come in different shapes, sizes, and materials such as alnico, ceramic, neodymium, and samarium cobalt.

For those interested in the scientific details of Gauss, it is a unit of magnetic induction in the centimeter-gram-second system of physical units. Gauss corresponds to the magnetic flux density that will induce an electromotive force of one abvolt in each linear centimeter of a wire moving laterally at one centimeter per second at right angles to a magnetic flux. One Gauss is equivalent to 10-4 tesla (T), the International System Unit, and is equal to one Maxwell per square centimeter. The Gauss unit was named after the German scientist Carl Friedrich Gauss.

Overall, Biomagnetism is a safe and non-invasive therapy that uses the power of magnets to help restore balance and harmony to the body's biochemistry.

Who discovered Medical Pair Biomagnetism?

The use of magnets for medicinal purposes has been known for centuries, but it was not until 1988 that Dr. Isaac Goiz Durán of Mexico City discovered a superior and efficient way of using magnets for health reasons. This discovery led to the birth of Medical Pair Biomagnetism, which is different from Magnet Therapy.

Medical Pair Biomagnetism involves the use of pairs of magnets to create a therapy with a theoretical scientific medical foundation that effectively diagnoses and treats disease. Biomagnetic practitioners are trained and expert in applying magnetic pairs (both negative and positive fields) with a focused mind, body, and spirit medical purpose. The objective of Medical Biomagnetism is to neutralize the biochemistry of the body by identifying and correcting specific pH distortions caused by microorganisms, intoxications, emotional issues, and other factors that cause illness.

In late 2015, Moses Durazo, BA, HHP, CBP, a biomagnetic pair therapy specialist with many years of experience, started thinking about how to best deliver a simple, effective self-care biomagnetic method. Durazo's Biomagnetic Recalibration System was designed to help individuals live the best possible version of their life by addressing mind, body, and spirit balance, as well as strategies for dealing with pain, detoxification, and boosting all body systems in order to maintain optimal wellness.

Durazo's findings, detailed in his book Biomagnetism: The Mind, Body, Spirit Recalibration System, evolved into a complete biomagnetic therapy program that individuals can do themselves (more information at *www.SaveMeMagnets.com*).

Is there scientific evidence?

Biomagnetism's power has been scientifically tested, and the results are compelling. In 2009, Dr. Isaac Goiz Durán and Dr. Raymond Hilu conducted a study that treated over two hundred patients with a variety of pathologies using Medical Biomagnetism. These patients had medical documents confirming their diagnoses and blood samples taken and analyzed before and after the biomagnetic session.

The results of the study were astonishing. The blood samples taken immediately after the biomagnetic session showed a significant improvement in circulation and oxygenation, with blood cells separated and moving around freely instead of clumped together. Furthermore, no traces of bacteria or fungus were found, and pH levels in the blood had shifted from acidosis to alkalosis in all cases without exception.

In addition to these objective improvements, patients reported subjective benefits such as pain relief and improved energy levels. And all of this was achieved with just a 20-minute biomagnetic session, compared to the months-long course of pharmaceuticals that would be required to achieve similar results using an allopathic medical approach.

It's important to note that Medical Biomagnetism is not a replacement for conventional medicine, but most certainly can be used in conjunction with allopathic treatment the majority of times. The results of this study provide strong evidence that Biomagnetism has significant potential to complement and enhance conventional medical treatments, offering patients a powerful tool for promoting healing and wellness.

Despite the fact that Dr. Goiz's diagnostic conclusions frequently differed from the patient's clinical allopathic diagnosis, Dr. Hilu emphasizes that the primary objective is to improve and cure patients, and the benefits of Biomagnetism speak for themselves. With its ability to balance the body's pH levels (erase potential hydrogen distortions), Biomagnetism offers a powerful new approach to health and healing that is well worth exploring.

Despite the evidence, why is there skepticism?

Despite the growing evidence of Medical Biomagnetism's effectiveness, there are still skeptics who question its validity. One reason for this skepticism may be due to the fact that Biomagnetism challenges the traditional Western allopathic medical model, which relies heavily on pharmaceuticals and surgery.

Additionally, some may dismiss Biomagnetism as a form of alternative or complementary medicine, which has a history of being viewed with suspicion by the medical establishment.

There may also be a lack of understanding or awareness about the scientific basis of Biomagnetism and how it works. It is important to note, however, that the scientific evidence supporting Biomagnetism is growing and more research is being conducted every day. It is also important to approach any new or alternative form of medicine with an open mind and to seek out reliable sources of information to make an informed decision about its use.

The difference between *Magnet Therapy, Medical Biomagnetism* and *Recalibration Biomagnetism?*

Magnet Therapy, Goizean Medical Biomagnetism, and Durazo's *Recalibration Biomagnetism* therapy all involve the use of magnets for healing, but they differ in their approach and philosophy.

Magnet Therapy is a broad term used to describe the use of magnets for healing, which includes various forms of therapy, such as static magnets, magnetic jewelry, and magnetic mattresses. The philosophy behind Magnet Therapy is based on the belief that magnets can improve blood flow, reduce inflammation, and alleviate pain. This approach generally places magnets on direct sites of pain and is not diagnostic nor does it address specific diseases or mind-spirit issues directly.

Goizean Medical Biomagnetism, on the other hand, is a specific type of biomagnetic therapy developed by Dr. Isaac Goiz Durán in Mexico in the 1980s. The philosophy behind Medical Biomagnetism is based on the idea that most illnesses are caused by pH imbalances in the body, which can be corrected by placing pairs of magnets on specific points on the body. The therapy is non-invasive, painless, and has no side effects, and has been used to treat a wide range of conditions, including infectious and chronic diseases.

Recalibration Biomagnetism therapy is another form of biomagnetic therapy developed by medical biomagnetic pair specialist, Moses Durazo. The therapy is based on the principle that the body has an energy field that can be affected by physical and emotional stressors, leading to imbalances that can cause illness. The therapy uses magnets to rebalance the body's energy field and restore health.

While Magnet Therapy and Biomagnetism are general terms used to describe various forms of therapies that use magnets or magnetic fields (static and electromagnetic), Goizean Medical Biomagnetism and Durazo's Biomagnetic Recalibration therapy are specific types of biomagnetic therapy that focus on correcting imbalances in the body to promote healing. Both therapies have gained popularity in recent years, and there is ongoing research to explore their efficacy and benefits.

BIOMAGNETIC SCIENCE AND PH- IMBALANCE-CAUSING FACTORS

TO FURTHER ELABORATE ON how Medical Biomagnetism works and how it can help your wellbeing, it's important to understand a few basic scientific chemical principles about our organism's composition.

In short, our complete body is mostly composed of the water molecule. The water molecule is comprised of two hydrogen and one oxygen atoms – the chemical formula being $H^{2}0$. Atoms are comprised of particles called neutrons, protons, and electrons; in other words, we are energy.

All chemical substances (water, vinegar, juice and so on) are measured on a potential hydrogen (pH) scale. In other words, all chemicals are evaluated to see if that substance is an acid or alkaline. Since we are mostly water, acidity and alkalinity of certain anatomical structures represent distortions and therefore an imbalanced organism that is not functioning optimally. When there are signs and symptoms in the body, it is certain that there are also pH imbalances.

When our biochemistry is pH neutral, meaning there is neither acidity nor alkalinity – 7.0 with a slight plus or minus variation – then our body is at its optimal energetic levels thus representing the proper biochemical balance as intended by nature, which leads to homeostasis, and thus self-regulation is optimized, which translates to a healthy organism that effectively protects and manages disease and illness causing factors.

Disease and illness causing factors cause specific pH imbalances of anatomical structures. These factors can be microorganisms such as viruses, bacteria, fungi, and parasites, organ or gland dysfunctions, intoxications, reservoirs, emotions stress, deficiencies and other...

When these microorganisms or other factors are present and impact our organism, they create both an acid and alkaline environment in specific anatomical structures of the body, which impairs the body's natural healing process. Biomagnetism works by identifying these specific pH distortions caused by microorganisms, toxins, emotional imbalances, and other, and using pairs of magnets to neutralize them.

The magnets act as tools to help restore balance to the body's pH levels, allowing the body to heal itself more effectively. This not only leads to an improvement in physical health, but it can also positively impact mental and emotional well-being, as the body's natural healing process is enhanced. By targeting specific pH imbalances in the body (organs, glands and other anatomical structures), Biomagnetism can help to prevent the development of chronic or degenerative diseases, while also supporting overall health and wellness.

What can Biomagnetism cure?

pH distortions can be caused by many factors such as microorganisms, toxins, emotional trauma, poor nutrition, and so on. Biomagnetism has the ability to identify and correct these specific pH distortions in the body, thereby addressing the root cause of the disease.

The range of conditions that can be treated with Biomagnetism is extensive and includes but is not limited to: infections, allergies, autoimmune diseases, endocrine disorders, respiratory conditions, gastrointestinal issues, neurological disorders, and musculoskeletal problems.

Even mental and emotional issues can be addressed with Biomagnetism because they too are related to biochemical imbalances in the body. It is important to note that Biomagnetism does not replace lifestyle habits. Biomagnetism works alongside other medical modalities, and nutrition to help the body heal and achieve optimal health.

What causes pH imbalances?

In addition to the factors mentioned above, there are also lifestyle choices that can contribute to pH imbalances, such as poor diet, lack of exercise, smoking, and alcohol and sugar intoxication and other.

It's important to note that while these factors can contribute to pH imbalances, not everyone who is exposed to them will develop a disease. Biomagnetism aims to identify and balance these pH imbalances before they develop into more serious conditions, but it's important to also make healthy lifestyle choices in order to maintain optimal health.

Furthermore, it's worth mentioning that emotional and spiritual health are often overlooked in conventional medicine, but can have a significant impact on overall wellbeing. Biomagnetism takes a holistic approach to healing, addressing not only physical symptoms but also emotional and spiritual imbalances that can contribute to disease.

What is a: virus, bacteria, fungus or a parasite?

It is important to understand the characteristics of each type of microorganism that can cause disease. Viruses are tiny infectious agents that cannot reproduce on their own, but they use a host cell to replicate and spread throughout the body. Some examples of viral infections include the flu, HIV, and hepatitis.

Bacteria are single-celled organisms that can cause a wide range of infections, such as strep throat, pneumonia, and tuberculosis.

Fungi are a type of microorganism that can cause infections of the skin, nails, and mucous membranes, such as athlete's foot, ringworm, and thrush.

Parasites are organisms that live on or inside another organism, known as the host, and can cause a variety of infections, such as malaria, lice, and tapeworms.

Each type of microorganism has its own unique characteristics, such as how it spreads, how it interacts with the body, and what biomagnetic pair treatments are effective against the specific pH distortions they cause. Therefore, accurate diagnosis and targeted biomagnetic treatment are crucial for successfully managing and eliminating these infections.

What are dysfunctions?

A dysfunction is an abnormality or impairment in the function of a specified bodily organ or system. For example, there are dysfunctions of glands (e.g. thyroids), organs (e.g. liver), or systems (e.g. nervous).

A pineal gland dysfunction, for example, can cause issues with sleep as well as a condition called vitiligo, where discoloration of the skin takes place.

Dysfunctions can have many underlying root causes such as infections. For example, suppose one has a horrible cold. The immune system terminates the infection, but because of this illness, the thyroid gland was left harmed and maybe caused a condition such as hyper-or-hypothyroidism. Another example of this would be the talk of "Long-COVID".

Other factors that can cause dysfunctions include poisoning from food sources like fructose or monosodium glutamate (MSG), which is a flavor enhancer used in many foods or energy drinks that put high stress on the body.

Manufacturers put countless numbers of preservatives in foods so they can keep them on the grocery shelves longer. All this adds up to wreak havoc with a body. The fact is that anything including emotional or behavioral alterations can cause a pH distortion, which can cause a dysfunction, disease and discomfort.

What are toxins?

Toxins are poisonous substances that can cause illness and even death. There are many sources for common toxins like environmental, fructose, foods, medicines, nutritional supplements, alcohol, drugs, pathogens, and so on. Many people consume toxins without understanding they are contributing to their own demise.

One of humanity's favorite poisons is fructose (generally referred to as sugar – although this is not a complete definition), but since it is so delicious, it is hard for many to believe or care about the overwhelming science that shows that it is detrimental to our health. (For more detailed information about the topic of sugar, view Dr. Robert Lustig's lectures and talks – viewable on YouTube).

In addition, pharmacists hand people information sheets that list side effects associated with their medication and yet people willingly take these questionable medications. Sometimes these pharmaceutical solutions are worse than the disease itself, and this can be seen today in the aftermath of the COVID vaccines rollout.

Others consume nutritional supplements thinking that because they are natural, then they must be good. This, however, is a false belief as one might be poisoning oneself by the chemical compounds used to make these supplements as well as offsetting the internal balance of vitamins and minerals. It is known that when the body has too much of one vitamin or mineral (or anything else, for that matter), this can inhibit the body's ability to assimilate other essential nutrients.

Pathogens (microorganisms) have their own metabolism, meaning they produce waste. To humanize this description, they *pee* and *poop* inside of us causing poisoning.

What is a psychological disorder?

A psychological disorder, also known as a mental disorder or mental illness, is a condition that affects a person's thinking, behavior, emotions, or mood in a way that significantly impairs their ability to function in daily life. Psychological disorders can range from mild to severe and can be caused by a variety of factors, such as genetics, environmental factors, life experiences, pH imbalance causing factors and other. Some examples of psychological disorders include depression, anxiety disorders, bipolar disorder, schizophrenia, personality disorders, and eating disorders.

What are emotional challenges?

Emotional challenges are difficulties that we encounter when managing and dealing with our emotions. Emotions are the result of biochemical hormonal responses, and there are many different emotions that we are capable of feeling, including *aggression, arrogance, greed, envy, fear, resentment, impatience, intolerance, hatred, doubt, guilt, loneliness*, and many more. It is essential to recognize and acknowledge these emotions, as they serve as signals to our bodies that something is not right.

The problem arises when we avoid unpleasant emotions and suppress them, leading to emotional challenges. These challenges can manifest in many ways, such as repeated negative patterns or placing blame on others. The key is to take responsibility for our actions and learn from our experiences to overcome these challenges.

Emotional challenges can also stem from traumas that were not dealt with at the time they occurred. These unresolved issues can affect our peace of mind and daily social functioning, leading to psychological and behavioral disorders, and of course, also create pH distortions. Emotional trauma has many root sources, but it is possible to overcome them. The use of both Medical Biomagnetism and Recalibration Biomagnetism can help us overcome these active emotional conflicts more easily by rebalancing our body's pH levels, and by providing a specific framework of introspection and Biomagnetism to follow.

It is essential to note that conscious or subconscious painful memories can affect our daily social functioning, and they may lead to psychological and behavioral disorders. Therefore, it is crucial to recognize and address these emotional challenges to maintain our mental and emotional health. We have free will to choose our behavior and make better choices, which can lead to a healthier and more fulfilling life.

What are deficiencies?

Deficiencies refer to the lack of essential nutrients that our body needs to function correctly, including minerals, vitamins, oils, water, and more. The most common reason for deficiencies is inadequate nutrition, where the foods we eat may not contain all the necessary nutrients or are affecting or microbiome. On top of this, another less obvious reason has to do with our body's pH balance.

When our body's pH level is distorted, it may have a difficult time absorbing the nutrients from the food we eat. In addition, excessive consumption of one particular mineral or vitamin can lead to distortions in the nutrient balance and inhibit the absorption of another nutrient, resulting in deficiencies.

Water is the most important nutrient that our body needs, and it is essential for all bodily functions. However, many people ignore water and opt for potentially toxic flavored drinks instead. Some people may even go to the opposite extreme and over-consume water, leading to mineral imbalances and other issues.

To maintain proper nutrient balance, it is crucial to consume a well-rounded diet that includes a variety of nutrient-rich foods, eliminate toxins, and incorporate Biomagnetism into your wellness care. Additionally, staying hydrated by drinking enough water throughout the day is essential.

What is spirituality and spiritual interference?

Spirituality is a complex and multifaceted concept that can vary greatly depending on one's beliefs and perspectives. At its core, spirituality relates to one's core beliefs and sense of connection to something greater than oneself, such as a higher power, God, or a creator. This can provide a sense of meaning and purpose in life, and can be an important aspect of one's overall well-being.

In addition to spiritual health, there is also the belief that spiritual entities, such as spirits or ghosts, exist and can interfere with our quality of life. While this is a controversial topic, some practitioners believe that these energies can impact our well-being. However, the belief in these entities and their impact on our health is not necessarily adopted by all practitioners.

Regardless of one's beliefs, it is important to honor nature's rules and strive to become a better version of ourselves each day. Following our intuition and acting from a place of goodness for all can lead to spiritual growth and overall well-being. It is also important to recognize that difficult times can often lead to great achievements.

When it comes to addressing spiritual interference, some practitioners use a non-invasive and non-religious approach to instruct these entities to leave. While this may seem unusual from a medical or scientific perspective, it is an example of how biomagnetic practitioners may apply science that is both proven and theoretical.

Ultimately, the topic of spirituality and spiritual interference is a sensitive one that should be approached with care and respect. If an individual feels that spiritual interference may be affecting them, they can discuss it with their practitioner and decide how best to address it.

What is a foreign DNA?

Foreign deoxyribonucleic acid (DNA) refers to genetic material that enters our bodies from sources outside of our own DNA. This can happen through blood transfusions, organ transplants, or other forms of medical intervention. While the idea that foreign DNA can alter personality or other traits is not widely supported by scientific evidence, there are some well-documented cases that suggest it is possible. For example, some people have reported changes in tastes for music, food, and sports after receiving transplants from donors who enjoyed those activities. In some rare cases, changes in blood type have been observed following a transplant.

For practitioners of Medical Biomagnetism and Bioenergetics, the challenge is to understand and identify to whom the disease process belongs during a treatment session. Is it the donor or the recipient who is reacting to bioenergetic questioning? While this field of study requires further research, it is important for patients to inform their practitioners if they have had blood transfusions or organ transplants.

What is a malignancy?

In Medical Biomagnetism and Bioenergetics, malignancy refers to a psycho-emotional interference related to negative emotions that another person has against us or vice versa. This interference can affect our peace of mind and wellbeing, keeping us in a state of emotional agitation. While it may not make scientific sense that someone's mental ill-wishes against another would alter that person's wellbeing when not directly voiced or demonstrated, the power of intention and energy can have an effect on us at the cellular level. Therefore, it is important for each of us to control negative thoughts against others for our collective well-being.

What are Chakra imbalances?

Chakras are energy vortexes that exist in the body and are believed to be connected to the glandular system. Imbalances in chakras can cause blockages, which can be corrected by helping the chakra(s) to balance itself using the power of intent through bioenergetic instruction. While there are different teachings about chakras, Dr. Goiz's approach is simple and effective in addressing chakra imbalances.

What is a reservoir?

A reservoir refers to a part of the body that contains harmful microorganisms that are not currently causing any symptoms of disease, but can become activated and cause an infection in the future. This can include areas such as organs, tissues, or bones. These microorganisms can remain dormant in the reservoir for an extended period of time, making it challenging to identify the source of an infection when symptoms do eventually arise. By identifying and addressing these reservoirs through the use of magnets and bioenergetic therapy, it is possible to prevent the activation of these harmful microorganisms and prevent the onset of disease.

How do you detect specific pH distortions?

The *biomagnetic* and *bioenergetic* approach are two different ways to detect specific pH distortions in the body during a medical biomagnetic session. A practitioner diagnosing biomagnetically places a magnet over 300 specific body parts, one at a time, while the patient lies face up on a therapy table. The reaction observed by the practitioner is either the shortening or lengthening of the right hemisphere if there is a pH distortion in that area. Leg or arm length can be measured to determine the reaction.

Bioenergetics, also known as muscle testing, can also be used to detect pH distortions, which yield the same shortening or lengthening reaction as the physical placement of a magnet.

What is Bioenergetics?

Bioenergetics is a method used by advanced biomagnetic practitioners to diagnose pH distortions of the organism and to address psychological, emotional, chemical, hormonal, and spiritual issues that cannot be addressed by Biomagnetism alone. It involves using the mind to communicate with the body's inner intelligence and reciting specific anatomy, emotional and psychological issues to detect any imbalances. The moment the leg length changes, it tells the practitioner where the magnet must be placed. Bioenergetics may also be referred to as muscle-testing or kinesiology by some healthcare practitioners, and it allows the practitioner to quickly scan the entire body in a few minutes as opposed to an hour using the biomagnetic method

While the idea of Bioenergetics may seem unusual and may cause skepticism in some, it has been shown to be effective over time. The reason why Bioenergetics works is because our DNA is capable of decoding and obeying the therapist's questions and commands, which allows the bioenergetics scan to be conducted in any language, even when the therapist and recipient are of different linguistic backgrounds.

For those interested in learning Bioenergetics for their personal use and understanding, there is a book titled "*Biomagnetism: The Mind, Body, Spirit Recalibration System*" which provides simple steps to gaining greater control of one's life.

Do I need to believe for it to work?

It is important to keep an open mind and be willing to try new things, especially when it comes to health and well-being. Believing in Biomagnetism is not necessary for the therapy to work, as scientific studies have shown measurable results from its application. However, if someone is skeptical or does not believe in the therapy, they may be less likely to try it or may not see the full benefit from it.

The *placebo* effect, where faith plays a role in healing, is also important to consider. Even in conventional medicine, the placebo effect is recognized as having a significant impact on treatment outcomes. Belief and positive thinking can have a powerful effect on our physical and mental health.

In addition to the placebo effect, it's important to consider the *nocebo* effect. This occurs when a person's negative expectations or beliefs about a treatment lead to negative outcomes, even if the treatment itself is neutral or beneficial. For example, if a person believes that Biomagnetism won't work for them, they may experience no improvement or even negative side effects, despite the treatment's potential effectiveness.

It's important for practitioners to address and acknowledge any negative beliefs or expectations that a patient may have, in order to minimize the potential for a nocebo effect. Practitioners should also provide clear information about the treatment and its potential benefits, in order to establish a positive and informed mindset in the patient.

Ultimately, the role of belief and mindset in the effectiveness of Biomagnetism and other treatments is complex and multifaceted. While belief and expectation may not be the sole determinants of treatment success, they do play a role and should be considered in the overall treatment approach.

SAFETY AND CONTRAINDICATIONS

MEDICAL BIOMAGNETISM HAS BEEN a safe and effective therapy for decades, as has some form of magnet therapy application that has been used for centuries. Magnetic energy is a natural force found throughout the planet and is safe for people of all ages and health conditions, including newborns. Unlike electromagnetic devices, Medical Biomagnetism does not involve electricity, so there is no risk of tissue burns or other injuries.

Unfortunately, the internet is full of misinformation about this natural therapy, which can make people hesitant to try it. For example, some articles claim that only the negative magnetic field should be used or that placing a magnet in the wrong location can make things worse. However, these claims are untrue.

It is also an inconvenient truth that mislabeled magnets are often used in the Medical Biomagnetic Pair field. This means that positive fields are labeled as negative, and vice versa. This fact does not pose a risk to anyone, but it does mean that the therapeutic benefits may not be as effective as possible.

To address common concerns and misconceptions about the safety of Biomagnetism, this chapter will provide answers to frequently asked questions. These include who should not use magnets, how to avoid potential risks, and what to do if you experience adverse effects.

How old must you be to try Medical Biomagnetism?

Medical Biomagnetism is an all-encompassing non-invasive therapy that supports the wellness of all life, making it a safe and natural option for individuals of all ages, from the beginning of life at conception, to newborn, the elderly and even those on their deathbed.

Is Biomagnetism safe for pregnant women?

Pregnant women can definitely benefit from Biomagnetism, but we would suggest starting Biomagnetism prior to pregnancy, so that both parents can already be in biochemical balance, resulting in optimal quality sperm and ovum and overall body function. Using Biomagnetism reduces the risk of complications during pregnancy, such as miscarriage, birth defects, stillbirth, premature birth, low birth weight, and passing infections to the baby, as well as other health conditions like asthma, diabetes, depression, eating disorders, epilepsy, high blood pressure, HIV, migraines, overweight or obesity, sexually transmitted infections, thyroid dysfunction, and uterine fibroids.

If a woman is already pregnant, Biomagnetism can still be beneficial as it can cause a healing and balancing reaction that is healthy for both mother and baby. Overall, Biomagnetism is a safe and natural therapy that can benefit anyone seeking to improve their health and well-being.

Is Biomagnetism safe while on chemotherapy or other treatments?

Biomagnetic therapy is generally safe and can be taken even if you are taking other pharmaceutical drugs or alternative medicines. However, if you are currently undergoing chemotherapy or have recently finished, it is essential to inform your biomagnetic therapist to determine whether it is appropriate for you or not at this particular time. Biomagnetism can amplify the effects of chemotherapy; by balancing your organism, it can cause cells to absorb more of the toxic pharmaceutical, which can be harmful.

Generally, people wait 2-3 months after the last chemotherapy session before undergoing medical biomagnetic therapy, but, a trained biomagnetic therapist will know when the time is right based on your unique condition. If you are undergoing chemotherapy or have recently finished, you may consider Recalibration Biomagnetism as the alternative, which are powerful self-care strategies, including a biomagnetic detoxification booster, which can help you process toxicity more efficiently (more information at www.SaveMeMagnets.com).

Is Biomagnetism painful?

Biomagnetism is not painful, if they did, perhaps children wouldn't love playing with magnets, or love going to Durazo's biomagnetic practice.

While some people may experience temporary discomfort during a session, it is usually due to the body adjusting itself, not the magnets or their strength. For example, people with tumors may feel slight discomfort at the tumor site, which usually lasts only a few minutes and is gone by the end of the session.

What happens when I mix Biomagnetism with allopathic treatment?

When it comes to mixing Biomagnetism with conventional allopathic treatments, there is generally no interference or negative effects. Biomagnetism can be used alongside other treatments to support the body's healing process. However, if you are taking medication, it is important to have a close working relationship with the prescribing doctor because biomagnetic therapy can help the body rebalance and heal, potentially reducing the need for medication or altering the dosage required.

Does Biomagnetism interfere with other natural therapies?

Biomagnetism is a safe and natural therapy that uses static magnets to balance the pH levels in the body and restore health. It is a complementary therapy that can be used alongside other natural therapies. In fact, combining Biomagnetism with other natural therapies can enhance the overall effectiveness of the treatments.

There is no evidence to suggest that Biomagnetism interferes with other natural therapies like acupuncture, alphabiotics, homeopathy, chiropractic, reflexology, and many others. These therapies all work to promote health and balance in the body, and they can work synergistically to help the body heal and restore itself.

Does Biomagnetism interfere with metallic surgical implants?

The presence of metallic surgical implants will not interfere with biomagnetic therapy. Implanted metals are non-ferrous, meaning they do not react to magnetism. In general, having surgical implants should not prevent a person from receiving the benefits of Biomagnetism therapy.

Does Biomagnetism interfere with pacemakers?

Biomagnetism does not interfere with pacemakers as long as precautions are taken. Pacemakers are electronic devices that are battery-powered, and they may be depleted by magnetic fields. However, biomagnetic therapy is safe for those with pacemakers as long as the magnets are not placed directly over the pacemaker.

It is important to inform your biomagnetic practitioner if you have a pacemaker. They will take precautions to ensure that the magnets are placed safely and do not interfere with the pacemaker. Magnets can be placed anywhere else on the body without any risk to the pacemaker.

WHAT TO EXPECT ON YOUR VISITS

BIOMAGNETISM IS A NATURAL, safe, and effective therapy that can help you achieve your specific health goals. It is a powerful and precise method that is 100% safe. To begin your journey towards better health, it is important to relax, be at peace, and envision your goals. Without knowing where you want to go, it's impossible to get there.

Each practitioner has their own methods, but during your first visit to Durazo Medical Biomagnetims' office, or seeking the MagnoGuide service (more about this later) these general steps are followed:

1. You become a member of the Private Membership Medical Association by signing a document.
2. You fill out a signs and symptoms questionnaire.
3. You have a brief interview with the practitioner assigned to you to address any questions or concerns.
4. You then lie comfortably, fully clothed, on a therapy table for approximately 40 minutes while the diagnosis and treatment take place.

What is the Private Membership Medical Association document?

The Private Membership Medical Association document is a legal agreement that you sign on your first visit at Durazo's practice, which makes you a member of the practice's private medical association.

The purpose of this document is to protect both the practitioner and the patient. In the United States, it is illegal for unlicensed individuals to diagnose and treat human conditions. By becoming a member of the private medical association, the practitioner can legally diagnose and treat conditions using Biomagnetism without fear of prosecution. The nominal one-time membership fee covers a lifetime membership and allows the patient to have access to treatments. Opting out of the membership is possible at any time. The Private Membership Medical Association document is necessary for the practice to legally provide biomagnetic therapy to the public in the United States.

What is the symptom questionnaire?

The symptom questionnaire is a simple form that you will be asked to fill out on your first visit to a biomagnetic practice. The purpose of the questionnaire is for you to list the main symptoms (if any) that are bothering you the most. This will help you keep track of changes in the intensity of your pain or discomfort.

You will rate the intensity of your symptoms on a 1-10 scale, which is helpful in tracking your progress. Although it is not necessary to share your symptoms, it is helpful in noticing changes. The biomagnetic process does not rely on symptomatology, allopathic diagnosis, or testing to determine where to place the magnets. However, reviewing the list of symptoms can help you understand if the pain or discomfort has significantly diminished or is gone. The symptom questionnaire is a useful tool to track your progress and see the level of improvement you are making.

What is the initial interview like?

During the initial interview, you will have a chance to talk about your symptoms with the practitioner assigned to you. This interview is an opportunity to ask questions about the therapy, discuss your body's functions, and set long-term health goals. Effective communication is essential for a successful partnership between you and your practitioner, and most biomagnetic practitioners value education and aim to keep you informed.

You can also ask your practitioner about their experiences working with people in situations similar to yours. If they get upset or defensive when you ask about their experience or qualifications, it could be a red flag, and you might want to consider finding another practitioner.

Durazo once had an experience of contacting a biomagnetic practitioner hoping to develop a working relationship with her. When he asked she had completed the advanced biomagnetic/bioenergetic training that Dr. Goiz offered at the time, she answered no. When asked if she would take the advanced training, she replied with a defensive response.

This experience highlights the importance of open communication and building trust based on the practitioner's professional experience. Overall, the initial interview is an opportunity to discuss your health goals and symptoms and establish a comfortable partnership with your practitioner.

How long are the sessions?

The length of biomagnetic sessions can vary depending on the geographic location and the patient's condition. The first visit is usually longer than subsequent visits, lasting about an hour or more due to paperwork and the initial interview.

Subsequent visits typically last about 40 minutes. The amount of time a person lies with magnets on their body varies based on the earth's latitude, with sessions in equatorial regions taking only 5-7 minutes, while in Southern California, a person typically keeps the magnets on their body for 27-30 minutes, and sometimes longer depending on planetary factors.

What if I can't lie down for a long time?

Some people may have conditions that make it difficult for them to lie down for extended periods of time, such as pregnancy or certain respiratory conditions. Others, like young children, will not lay still for the complete duration of the treatment.

In these cases, the practitioner can work with the patient to find a comfortable position that allows for treatment. With children, Durazo tapes small, yet powerful magnets to their body, which allows them to move about freely. The goal is to make the member as comfortable as possible while still receiving the benefits of Biomagnetic therapy.

Can somebody come with me to my appointment?

Durazo's practice encourages you to bring someone to support you and ensure your peace of mind during the biomagnetic therapy session. This educational experience can benefit everyone involved. However, it is crucial that you bring someone who fully supports the process, as having someone in the room who is there to inspect and criticize can interfere with the intended peaceful and healthful experience.

What will I feel during the biomagnetic session?

During a biomagnetic session, some people may feel sensations caused by the magnetic field, while others may not feel anything at all. Reports of experiences during a session may include digestive noises, twitching, tingling, temporary pain, hot or cold sensations, vivid colors, or unexpected memories and emotions. Although these sensations may occur during a session, it is important to remember that it is a healing response, not a worsening of symptoms.

What did you find? What's wrong with me?

Biomagnetic practitioners aim to correct pH imbalances in the body, which are often the cause of pain and suffering. However, how a practitioner answers the question of *"What's wrong with me?"* may depend on legal considerations, particularly in unlicensed medical fields.

If a practitioner is protected by a private membership association, such as in Durazo's practice, they may be able to provide a more detailed explanation of the pH imbalances and infections (or other) that the magnets are addressing. On the other hand, if the practitioner is not licensed or protected, they may provide a more general explanation, such as the root of the health issues being biochemical imbalances.

How did I get this condition/infection/problem?

As discussed previously, in Biomagnetism the main objective is to correct the pH imbalances that have resulted from infections and other factors. While a practitioner may identify an obvious source of the infection, such as exposure to pets, there may be other less apparent sources such as consuming contaminated food or touching contaminated surfaces.

Additionally, infections can also be transmitted through air, sexual contact, and other means. Microorganisms are ubiquitous and impossible to completely avoid. Emotional stress can also weaken the body and create an environment for microorganisms to thrive. Some infections can even be inherited from parents during conception or birth. While it is important to understand the cause of the condition or infection, the primary goal of Biomagnetism is to restore pH balance and promote overall health.

What will I feel after the biomagnetic session?

After a medical biomagnetic session, people generally feel three different ways: 1. It is obvious to them that they feel better, for example, less pain or increased energy, 2. Others may experience a healing crisis and may feel tired and sleepy, and 3. They may not be certain about what they feel; some simply do not have enough awareness or appreciation about their shifts. For example, sometimes people say, *"I didn't really feel any shifts"*, but upon further probe, they will reveal, for example, that they sleep better, are in a better mood, which all of these things are really big things.

What is a healing crisis?

A healing crisis is a temporary worsening of symptoms that may occur after a biomagnetic therapy session. It is also known as a detox reaction or a Herxheimer reaction. It is a common, normal and expected response to the therapy, as the body eliminates toxins and restores balance; however, it is not perceivable to everybody.

Examples of signs or symptoms that may occur during a healing crisis include:

- Increased fatigue
- Headaches

- Nausea
- Flu-like symptoms
- Skin rashes
- Digestive issues (diarrhea, constipation, gurgling stomach)
- Mood swings
- Joint pain
- Sweating
- Increased urination

It is important to note that not everyone experiences a healing crisis, and if it does occur, it is usually mild and short-lived. It is a sign that the body is undergoing a positive change, and the symptoms should resolve on their own within a few days to a few weeks.

What if I don't feel anything after my session?

If you don't feel anything different after a biomagnetic session, it's possible that you're not consciously aware of any changes happening in your body. Sometimes those around us may notice that we are complaining less, have more energy, or are more active, even if we don't consciously realize it ourselves. It's also possible that pain has disappeared without us even realizing it.

However, it's important to note that some people do feel things during a session but may still feel like nothing has happened. For example, a person may feel their headache disappear and feel better breathing, but still be hesitant to schedule another appointment because they are unsure if the therapy is really working for them.

If you're not noticing any shifts in your body or mind after a session, it may be helpful to perform a self-evaluation process to help you become more aware of any changes. You can learn more about this process and how to perform self-care biomagnetic recalibration on yourself using Durazo's Biomagnetic Recalibration System.

However, if you have tried performing Biomagnetism on yourself and still don't experience any shifts, it's a good idea to seek out a trained medical biomagnetic pair therapist. The next chapter will talk about how you can access Biomagnetism from anywhere in the world.

What should I do after a session?

After a biomagnetic session, it is important to take care of yourself and continue living a healthy life that supports your well-being. In general, an immediate action to take is to either disinfect or get a new toothbrush and razor blade as these items can contain microorganisms that may re-infect you.

Listen to your body and intuition. If you feel tired, rest. If you feel energized, exercise. If you feel hungry, eat balanced and healthy food. It is important to keep yourself hydrated as this may help diminish the intensity of any possible detoxifying effects.

It is also important to that your partner, spouse and household members be treated as well, even if they are not showing any symptoms, as we can transfer microorganisms to one another without being aware. As a whole, make maintaining wellness a daily habit, simply by making the time to identify areas in your life that can be improved and take action towards achieving a better quality of life. Remember to dedicate every moment of your life to achieving your dreams and vision for a perfect life.

Also, check out Durazo's other books to gain simple yet powerful strategies to help guide you in improving your life, including the use of SaveMeMagnets.com's self-care biomagnetic kits.

SPECIAL SERVICES: MAGNO-GUIDE AND DISTANCE HEALING

THE ACCESSIBILITY OF MEDICAL Biomagnetism has long been a concern for those seeking effective treatment. With only a handful of practitioners worldwide, this therapy has remained largely unknown and misunderstood by the majority of the world's population. Moreover, traditional in-person sessions with certified practitioners have made it difficult for those in remote areas or with limited mobility to access this treatment. But, thanks to Moses Durazo's ***MagnoGuide*** service, Medical Pair Biomagnetism is now accessible to anyone, anywhere.

The MagnoGuide service is a cutting-edge health service that combines the power of Medical Biomagnetism with the convenience of modern technology. Moses Durazo and his growing team of expert biomagnetic practitioners have developed a unique program to provide you with the guidance and support you need to achieve optimal health and wellness.

How does the MagnoGuide work?

To get started, simply purchase the service through *SaveMeMagnets.com*, and you'll receive an email with instructions on how to send in basic information about yourself, including your name, date of birth, geographic location, symptoms, and any other relevant health history details.

Next, Moses Durazo, or another certified biomagnetic specialist will review your information and create a personalized treatment plan specifically for you. This plan will include a diagram indicating where to place the magnets on your body for optimal results.

Please note that for this MagnoGuide service, you'll need a set of magnets. It's essential to use the SaveMeMagnets.com brand to ensure that you have correctly labeled magnets.

Once you receive your personalized illustration, you can begin your treatment right away. It's incredibly easy to use, and you don't need any prior knowledge or experience with Medical Biomagnetism to benefit from it. All you need to do is follow the instructions and place the magnets on your body as directed, right in the comfort of your own home.

Why should you start using the MagnoGuide?

The MagnoGuide offers numerous benefits for those seeking to improve their health and wellbeing:

- **Convenience**: access your health program from anywhere, at any time
- **Personalized attention**: connect with your biomagnetic practitioner for individualized support and guidance
- **Affordability**: our program is available at a fraction of the cost of in-person biomagnetic therapy (no travel or time off from work)
- **Easy to use**: our program is designed to be user-friendly and accessible to individuals of all ages and backgrounds
- **Effective**: Biomagnetism has been shown to be a powerful tool for improving health and wellbeing, with countless success stories from individuals who have used this therapy

Don't let chronic pain and illness hold you back from living your best life. Start using MagnoGuide today and experience the power of biomagnetism for yourself.

What is Distance Healing?

Distance Healing, also known as *Remote Healing*, is a technique used in biomagnetic practices to treat someone who is not present physically. This means that anyone can receive the benefits of Biomagnetism without stepping outside of their home or being in the same room as the practitioner.

Distance Healing has been documented by medical professionals as far back as the mid-1900s, and it is based on the idea that the entire universe is interconnected, and nothing exists on its own. Using Biomagnetism and Bioenergetics, distance healing is just as effective as if the person were physically present.

A distance healing session is done by placing magnets on a surrogate, who directs their consciousness and intention to address the recipient's health. A distance healing session is *only* performed when the recipient requests it or consents to it. It is important to note that a distance healing session can be performed with children if the parents request it, and a family member can make the decision for someone in a coma or who cannot communicate.

Can I treat my pet with Biomagnetism?

Yes, it is possible to treat your pets with Biomagnetism. The most convenient way to do this is to treats pets via Distance Healing. Again, this method involves placing magnets on a surrogate, directing consciousness and intention to address the pet's health.

If you were thinking of using the MagnoGuide as a pet service, this is possible; however, you are faced with the challenge of securing the magnets in specific areas.

THE BIG ISSUES

WHEN CONSIDERING ALTERNATIVE THERAPIES such as Biomagnetism, there are often many questions that come to mind. Here are some BIG issue frequently asked questions regarding biomagnetic treatment and their answers.

Can you guarantee a cure?

As with any medical treatment, there are no guarantees of a cure. Biomagnetism can support the body's natural healing process, but results may vary depending on individual circumstances. It is important to have realistic expectations and work with a trained biomagnetic therapist to develop a treatment plan that works best for you. With the MagnoGuide or Distance Healing service, you can have access to Durazo and his team of professional therapists regardless of where you are in the world.

How many sessions do I need?

The number of sessions needed varies depending on the individual's condition and response to treatment. Some people may experience improvement after just one session, while others may need four or more sessions to see significant improvement. When Medical Biomagnetism is used for maintenance, meaning there are no existing health challenges, at the bare minimum, should be applied once per year; fitness-minded individuals tend to seek it once per quarter (four times per year) or at the first sign of any discomfort.

From a self-care perspective using Recalibration Biomagnetism, you can use it on a daily basis. There is no such thing as overdosing because it is safe, natural and non-pharmaceutical.

How much does it cost, and does insurance pay for it?

As of 2023, insurance does not cover Medical Biomagnetism, at least not in the USA. However, individuals seeking biomagnetic services can file claims with their insurer to increase awareness and the possibility of reimbursement. The cost of Medical Biomagnetism varies depending on the practitioner and location, with some practitioners adopting a sliding scale, as Durazo does. Generally, treatment fees are similar to those of other natural medicine practitioners. For accurate pricing information, it is advisable to contact a certified biomagnetic practitioner directly.

Should I go to the hospital or do Biomagnetism first?

If you are experiencing a serious or life-threatening situation, seek professional help right away; Biomagnetism is not a replacement for emergency medical treatment. Once you have been evaluated and treated by a medical doctor for the emergency situation, then you may use Biomagnetism in conjunction with allopathic treatment as previously discussed. If you or loved one will not be discharged any time soon, the MagnoGuide or Distance Healing services are suggested.

Do you prescribe medication or supplements?

Biomagnetic therapy does not typically involve the prescription of medication or supplements, unless the practitioner is licensed to do so or has a supplementing branch within their practice. It is common for individuals to wonder how they can get better without taking pills, as our society has ingrained the idea that health is found in medication. However, in Biomagnetism, the magnetic field serves as the medicine that balances the body's pH levels and promotes homeostasis, which ultimately supports the body's natural healing process. Recalibration Biomagnetism can be likened to an over-the-counter supplement. Unlike traditional medicine that relies on pills, Biomagnetism focuses on using the body's natural energy to promote wellness.

Should I stop taking medication or supplements?

Ultimately, the decision to start or stop taking medication or supplements is up to you. During the biomagnetic diagnostic process, it is possible for the practitioner to detect any potential intoxication from pharmaceuticals or supplements. Through bioenergetics, the practitioner can also determine the optimal dosage of medication or supplement that would be most beneficial for you. However, it is important to emphasize that the decision to continue or discontinue any medication or supplement should be made by you, in consultation with your healthcare provider(s). The biomagnetic practitioner can provide valuable information to help you make an informed decision, but the ultimate responsibility for your health lies with you.

Are there people who cannot be helped?

Although Biomagnetism has been demonstrated to effectively treat a broad range of health conditions, there are instances where the level of improvement may be limited. While Biomagnetism is appropriate for almost everyone since the science is advantageous, a more relevant query would be to ask how much it can benefit you.

It is also essential to question how much you are contributing to your health problems through your actions and inactions. If the biomagnetic practitioner identifies a wellness action to take around nutrition or emotions, would you be willing to follow through with it? It's critical to remember that Biomagnetism is just one aspect of the multi-dimensional components required for attaining and maintaining optimal health and wellness.

Can I put magnets on myself?

Yes, you can put magnets on yourself with the proper knowledge, training or guidance. As previously mentioned, the MagnoGuide service shows you exactly where to place the magnets on your body to receive the benefits of Medical Biomagnetism from wherever you are located in the world – all you need is magnets, and the SaveMeMagnets.com® brand is suggested.

Also, the Recalibration Biomagnetism strategies were designed specifically to empower individuals to perform on themselves. You may receive proper training and education through courses available on the website www.SaveMeMagnets.com. One such resource is the 6-Day Recalibration Challenge, which is an online program that provides step-by-step guidance on how to perform Recalibration Biomagnetism on yourself. The program includes video tutorials, live Q&A sessions, and support from biomagnetic specialist Moses Durazo to help you get the most out of your magnet therapy self-care practice.

It is important to note that while using magnets on yourself can be safe and effective, it is still recommended to seek the advice of a qualified healthcare practitioner for any serious or chronic health conditions.

BONUS SELF-CARE STRATEGY: THREE MAGNETS FOR PAIN RELIEF

HERE IS A HIGHLY effective pain/tumor relief protocol that you can perform on yourself using the biomagnetic techniques of the Recalibration System, more specifically the book, *Biomagnetism: The Mind, Body, Spirit Recalibration System.*

You can obtain the health magnets required for this protocol at *www.SaveMeMagnets.com.* This safe and natural alternative to addictive painkillers has helped many clients relieve and even eliminate pain. However, it is important to note that this biomagnetic combination is not a substitute for medical care.

It is also important to remember that some users may experience a temporary increase in pain while using this protocol. This is a positive sign that transformation is taking place, and the pain will likely diminish or disappear after a few minutes.

Suggested for:

- *Physical Trauma*: the negative field on cuts, scratches, sprains, strains, bruises, fractures, broken bones, or other.
- *Localized Pain, Tumors/Growths*: the negative field on the site of pain or problem area.
- *Lacking Concentration:* the negative field on forehead or cerebral area where damage, if any, is defined.

- *Blood Sugar Levels: the* negative field on pancreas

Time Duration: 30 minutes each application, at least twice per day, until present issue improved or as needed. Because this formula can be used for maintenance, for example, maintaining mental focus, use at least twice per week for self-care maintenance.

Mindful Intention: The intention is to release and let go of pain and/or to bring balance to a specific body part.

Question: *What mind, body, spirit actions and inactions are contributing to this pain?* The reason this question is important is so that you may consider possible lifestyle actions that are contributing to this pain, and when possible, shift those behaviors and/or find ways to counter the effects of the behavior(s). For example, a repetitive work action (or inaction such as prolonged sitting) may cause stiffness; therefore, this awareness my bring focus into an action such as stretching or other.

To use this trio formula:

1. Place a positive magnet on the left kidney,
2. Another positive magnet on the right kidney, and
3. A negative magnet on the area of pain or tissue growth.

*Please note that when a positive or negative magnet is placed on a specific area, it means that the corresponding field is the one that touches your body, or in other words, it is the side that faces towards your body.

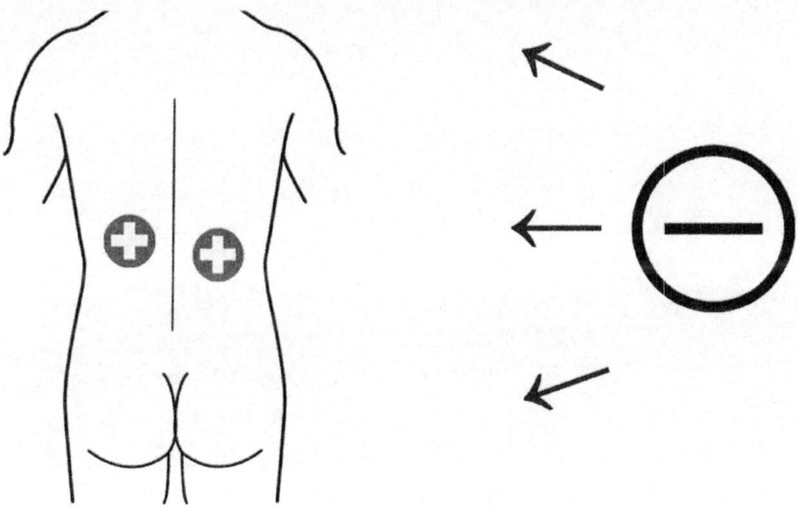

CONCLUSION

THE INFORMATION PRESENTED IN this FAQs book has the power to save lives and improve the quality of life for everyone. Goizean Medical Pair Biomagnetism, Bioenergetics and Recalibration Biomagnetism are safe, powerful, practical, precise, and effective scientific methods that everyone should be using regularly. Don't wait until something hurts to seek therapy, diseases can enter our body silently and sometimes only detected when it's too late.

We all deserve to function with optimal energy levels and Biomagnetism can help us achieve that. Even if you think you are fine, you can still enhance the quality of your life and that of your family members by incorporating Biomagnetism into your routine, whether you seek in-person services, remote or online services such as Biomagnetic Distance Healing, the MagnoGuide or Recalibration Biomagnetism.

To take your knowledge and practice of Biomagnetism to the next level, consider taking courses and purchasing kits. Another book in this series, *Biomagnetism: The Mind, Body, Spirit Recalibration System*, provides complete instructions and diagrams for a full recalibration of your body to achieve optimal well-being. And for the health magnets needed to perform your recalibration, visit www.SaveMeMagnets.com.

Don't wait any longer to experience the incredible benefits of Biomagnetism in your life!

ABOUT THE AUTHOR MOSES DURAZO

MOSES DURAZO IS A Certified Biomagnetic Practitioner (CBP) and Holistic Health Practitioner (HHP) based in Orange County, California. He is a strong advocate for the alternative medicine industry and has authored several books.

Durazo's journey to becoming a biomagnetic practitioner is a fascinating one. He began his studies by interning as a Medical Assistant at the University of California Irvine Medical Clinic and later served as a research assistant at the Center for AIDS Prevention Studies (CAPS) at the University of California San Francisco and Children's Hospital of Los Angeles. However, it was his exposure to holistic healthcare during his undergraduate studies at the University of California Santa Cruz that caused a paradigm shift in his way of thinking. He completed UCSC's holistic health practitioner certification program and graduated with a Bachelor of Arts in Language Studies.

After graduation, Durazo traveled extensively throughout Europe, Asia, and Latin America, gaining a broader perspective on the struggles people face in obtaining and maintaining optimal mind, body, and spiritual balance. In 2008, a trip to Mexico piqued his curiosity about Goizean Medical Biomagnetism as a specific healthcare therapy. He studied with Dr. Isaac Goiz Durán in Mexico City and was amazed by the healing results he witnessed.

Durazo's personal experience with chronic health issues led him to believe that pioneering this science would be his mission.

He also trained in Alphabiotic (Spinal) Alignments. To learn more about Moses Durazo and his wellness mission, please visit www.SaveMeMagnets.com

WORKS CITED

Britannica, E. (2014). *Britannica.com*. Retrieved 2014, from http://www.britannica.com/EBchecked/topic/227199/gauss.

Cayce, E. (2014). *http://www.edgarcayce.org/are/edgarcayce.aspx*. Retrieved from http://www.edgarcayce.org/are/edgarcayce.aspx.

CBS. (2014, October 5). 60 Minutes.

Goiz Durán, D. I. (2008). *El Fenómeno Tumoral.* 3rd Edition: Universidad Autónoma Chapingo.

Goiz Durán, D. I. (2008). *El Par Biomagnético.* Universidad Autónoma Chapingo.

Goiz Durán, D. I., & Hilu, D. R. (2009). *Par biomagnético hongos, virus, bacterias y parásitos.* Oxford International University.

Greene, B. (2011). NOVA-beta. http://www.pbs.org/wgbh/nova/physics/spooky-action-distance.html, PBS.

Centers for Disease Prevention and Control (CDC). http://www.cdc.gov/features/antibioticresistancethreats/

September 17, 2014

Printed in Great Britain
by Amazon

53083369R00040